Healing the DNA

How Generational Iniquities Affect Genetic Disorders

Dr. Pat Legako & Dr. Dee Legako

Published by:

Jubilee
Resources International Inc.
Equipping Christians, Liberating Captives
www.JubileeResources.org

Original published notes were entitled "Smart Bomb" Prayers.

Additional copies of this book are available from:

Jubilee Resources International Inc.

PO Box 3, Feilding 4740, New Zealand

or our secure Internet Webshop at

www.jubileeresources.org

All art work was created by Linda Kukuk, Pat's sister.

ISBN 978-1-87746388-4

CONTENTS

About Dee and Pat Legako:

They have been married for 46 years and have a grown son, Kevin, a daughter-in-law, Yuki, one granddaughter, Gabrielle and one grandson, Ansel.

With an understanding of genetic diseases, mental health and spiritual warfare, Dee and Pat bring a unique viewpoint to bear on the healing and deliverance of people suffering from schizophrenia and other genetically-based diseases.

Dee serves as an elder and board member for Church on the Rock, Oklahoma City. He is a graduate of Oklahoma State University with a B.S. in Premedical Science and University of Oklahoma with a medical degree. He served as a flight surgeon in the United States Air Force. He served on the Edmond Youth Council for ten years as well as serving on the Board of Directors for the Edmond Hope Center for ten years and the Board of Directors for Vine Life Ministries for three years. He currently volunteers his time as a Clinical Associate Professor with the Department of Family Medicine for the University of Oklahoma. He is a board certified Family Physician with a busy medical practice in Edmond, Oklahoma.

Pat leads the deliverance ministry team for Church on the Rock, Oklahoma City. A registered nurse, Pat spent years stuffing her medical knowledge into the back of her mind so she could pray in faith. It wasn't until the first time Doris Wagner asked her to minister to a schizophrenic that she began to realize that God had uniquely qualified her to do so. She has a Doctorate degree in Practical Ministry from Wagner Leadership Institute. A member of the Apostolic Round Table of the International Society of Deliverance Ministers, Pat speaks and ministers at regional and national conferences and has completed her first book project, with co-author, Cyndi Gribble, *"Deliverance, Rescuing God's People."*

Foreword

Having taught in their church, having stayed in their home, and having seen the fruit of their ministry, I can vouch for the solid medical and Biblical foundations of this couple. I was present when Pat first taught this subject at the annual conference of the ministry we both serve on the Apostolic Council of, and I immediately recommended them to put this information in to print. They asked my assistance in doing that, which I was thrilled to arrange.

Pat and Dee's goal is to see people healed and made whole. Knowing them for well over a decade has given me a respect and admiration for this couple.

You can use their material with confidence.

Selwyn R. Stevens, Ph.D. (Bib.St); D.Min.

President: Jubilee Resources International Inc.

(Note: Pat recently passed to her eternal reward. Dee continues his work.)

Introduction

The purpose of writing this book is to introduce the reader to the basics of genetics and how to create "smart bomb prayers" for the healing of genetic based disorders and diseases.

The field of genetics is developing at such a rapid pace that it is impossible to write prayers based on genetic research today that will be relevant next year. Therefore, our goal is to equip the reader with a model for writing such prayers as the need arises.

The book is written in the first person by Pat Legako for ease of reading, but Dee has contributed equal input. When Pat brought the research she had gathered on genetics and asked for his help, he patiently spent hours with her sorting through the material to glean what would be helpful. He meticulously brought her up to date on the study of genetics and helped her understand what they had discovered. Dee wrote the prayers that you will find in chapter six of this book and helped Pat prepare a presentation for teaching the material.

Chapter One

The Beginning

In the mid 1980s my husband and I left a denominational church in search of more. We ended up in a church that taught the Bible as God's Word. Two years after that we found a Bible study that was taught by John Benefiel, who was a stock broker and certified financial planner and is now our pastor. He also taught the Bible as God's Word that should be obeyed, and this began an incredible journey in growth for us. I ran into a little problem, however, when it came to believing for healing. I am a registered nurse and my husband is a medical doctor. I have always worked in hospitals with very sick patients and I had a mind-set that certain disease processes were terminal, some were not curable but treatable and some were curable.

I had no problem praying in faith for finances, jobs, studies, etc. but when it came to healing some things were terminal! I knew this was wrong so I set about correcting it. The only thing I could do, at first, was ask people not to tell me the diagnosis, just ask me to agree with them for healing of a serious disease. I could stand with them if I didn't know that what we were praying for was on my "list of terminal illnesses."

Later I learned to stuff my medical knowledge into a compartment labelled "work related." I could pull out my faith and pray for any condition as long as I didn't think about it medically. I don't know of any inherited disease that is curable.

When I was asked to pray for a young man with schizophrenia, I cried out to God and asked Him, *"How am I going to do this?"* His answer surprised me. *"Study the genetics of schizophrenia,"* He said. This completely messed up my compartments! It was time for a paradigm shift. As I made this shift a wonderful thing happened, I learned to use diagnoses as prayer points.

Chapter Two
Grady's Story

In 2002, several members of my deliverance team and I were doing altar ministry at an out-of-state conference when Dr. Doris Wagner sent a woman to me. The woman's son, whom I'll call Grady, had been newly diagnosed with schizophrenia. He began exhibiting symptoms when he was thirteen years old. He was now fifteen and appeared to be heavily medicated. The teenager's behavior was reminiscent of my case study patient, also a schizophrenic, during my psychiatric rotation in nursing. Grady refused to meet my gaze.

"I'm sorry. I can't look at you," he said, staring at the floor. *"The computer chip in my head that I got from the TV will hurt you if I look at you."* His speech was slurred.

"She's dead. She's dead," he murmured.

"Who's dead?" One of my team asked.

"She was with me, but now she's dead," he answered.

John Eckhardt had just led the entire conference in mass deliverance. Clearly, he had been delivered from a demonic entity that had held him in bondage. The only way he could express it was, *"She's dead"*.

This woman desperately wanted help for her son, but as I looked around the room I realized that we had to vacate the building in fifteen minutes so they could set up for a wedding. There wasn't time.

"I can't help you," I told the mother, hating to dash the hope I saw in her eyes. She reminded me of the woman recorded in Matthew 15: 22-28, who begged Jesus to deliver her demon-possessed daughter. I paused. *"But if you can come to Oklahoma for a few days we'll be happy to pray for your son."*

She agreed to make the trip.

Case History

Grady is the second child in a family of four boys. None of the other children have exhibited symptoms of schizophrenia, however the oldest brother had exhibited symptoms of rage, anger, ADD and 'supposed'

Bipolar Disorder … much of which abated with changes in nutrition. Grady began talking normal baby talk around eleven or twelve months of age, but he stopped at fourteen months. He didn't talk again until he was three years old, but his speech was so garbled that only his mother could understand him. From age three through the sixth grade, he received speech therapy twice a week. He progressed so slowly in first grade that his parents decided to hold him back. By fourth grade he couldn't keep up with the other students, and his teacher suggested he be tested.

Grady was diagnosed with attention deficit disorder and central auditory processing deficit. With his teachers working to accommodate these learning disabilities, he improved and finished fourth, fifth and sixth grades. The grade school he attended was a small one where all the teachers knew all the students.

Grady's mother suspected that the transition from a small grade school to a bustling middle school eight times larger would be a difficult adjustment for him. But the adjustment never occurred. With each passing week of his seventh grade year, Grady became more confused, disoriented and fearful, finally withdrawing into a world of his own. His teachers suggested that Grady be treated by a local psychiatrist who wanted to admit him for observation. When his mother refused to allow inpatient care, he was enrolled in outpatient group and individual counseling sessions every day after school. Four months later his condition had deteriorated. He finished seventh grade having been diagnosed with depression, bipolar disorder, attention deficit disorder, and social anxiety disorder. Doctors prescribed an antidepressant.

Within four days of beginning the antidepressant, Grady was almost catatonic making it next to impossible to interact with him. On two separate occasions, he wandered away from the family and got lost. His mother discontinued the medication.

The rest of the summer became a vigil to keep him safe. On one occasion he asked for a match. When questioned why he needed it Grady showed his mother the torch he was making. It consisted of rolled newspaper inserted in a glass bottle filled with gasoline.

During eighth grade Grady's schoolwork was nonexistent. As his paranoia escalated, he hid in the school's bathrooms or janitor's closet to avoid the *"stares of all those people talking about me."* Eventually the school provided a para-professional to meet Grady at the door and sit beside him in class. By November of that year, the school insisted he receive help. Under pressure, Grady's mother allowed him to be admitted to the hospital for psychiatric testing and observation. He was diagnosed with schizophrenia and put on anti-psychotic medications. His mother learned that statistically the rate of recovery from childhood schizophrenia was only five percent, and usually involved 20 years of medication and institutionalization.

Grady went back to school but not for full days. His hygiene suffered and the medication caused him to gain weight so rapidly that his skin tore. His family begged the doctor to change the medication. With the medication change, his condition deteriorated so rapidly that Grady asked to be hospitalized. The hospitalization lasted five weeks. While in the hospital, demonic spirits began interacting with Grady. One spirit introduced itself as a "Cop." One of the spirits sometimes spoke to him as a male, Michael. At other times it spoke as a female, Michelle.

Home from the hospital, school consisted of three hours in a small room working one-on-one with a para-professional. In May of that year Grady's mother took him to the deliverance conference where we met.

Praying for Direction

It was seven months from the first time I met Grady and his mother until they arrived in Oklahoma. During that time my team and I fasted and prayed, asking for God's direction. As I prayed, the Lord told me not to look up any case studies on schizophrenia. Clearly, He didn't want my faith to do a nosedive from reading them. What He told me to do surprised me. ***"Study the genetics of schizophrenia,"*** He said.

From my college education, I had only the most basic understanding of genetics, pretty much limited to recessive and dominant genes for eye color. But in recent years the U.S. Human Genome Project had identified approximately 80,000 genes in human DNA, determined the sequence of the three billion base pairs that make up human DNA, and stored the information in databases.

Clearly there is a genetic element to schizophrenia, as the tendency for the disease can be passed from parent to child, although it is generally triggered by stress. As I printed off page after page of genetic research on schizophrenia, I realized God had directed me to a gold-mine of information.

The research was so technical that I had trouble deciphering it, so I sat down to review it with my husband, Dee, a medical doctor. *"Imagine the human genome as a library,"* he said, explaining it in the simplest of terms. *"The chromosome is a book in the library. The band on each chromosome is a chapter in the book. Each gene is a sentence, and each base pair is a letter."* I was getting the picture.

As Dee read through the research, he got excited. *"The chromosome affected in schizophrenia is 22Q11,"* he said. *"The problem occurs where the protein is attached to the chromosome. In this case it's a gene called PRODH2. This is how the generational curse is passed down. The iniquity damages the chromosome, which is passed down in damaged form to the next generation through the blood!"*

We stared at one another in stunned silence. No wonder God told me to study the genetics of the disease. Now we could make a plan.

As I met with Dee and our team members, we realized that for Grady to get well, we had to treat him in three distinct ways. The first way was through deliverance. The second thing he needed was healing of his gene PRODH2 and the chromosome 22Q11. In addition, Grady needed behavior modification to teach him new ways to cope. Grady's mother and her friend who came with them for prayer support would both need deliverance as well as a written plan for after care.

We got to work developing our strategy. I assigned three teams of two people each - one to work with the mother, one to work with the friend, and another to work with Grady. I assigned myself to the mother. I assigned a team of sisters to Grady. One of them, Dee Dee Roberts, flows very powerfully in the prophetic and in spiritual warfare and leads the adolescent deliverance ministry in our church. The other, Dawnetta Russell, heads up our children's deliverance ministry. She has a master's degree in psychology and worked in the mental health field for eight years doing psychotherapy as well as teaching abnormal and developmental psychology at the college level. Today she is a high school counselor for high risk teens. While Dee Dee primarily handles the spiritual warfare, Dawnetta specializes in behavior modification.

The medical pair of the team, my husband and I, worked together to write specific prayers for healing each abnormality known to be associated with schizophrenia. Since some theories suggest that schizophrenia may be caused by a retrovirus, we tried to cover all the bases in the prayer which is included in chapter six of this book.

As time for Grady's deliverance drew near I presented our plans and the prayers we'd written to my pastor, Dr. John Benefiel, for his input and prayer. I also told Grady's mother that I could not do the deliverance unless Grady's pastor gave his permission for us to proceed. We had a long phone conversation, and he approved our plan and prayed for us as well.

A Step of Faith

In July of 2002, Grady, his mother, and her friend arrived in Oklahoma for three days. Although each of them was ministered to in the same location, neither Grady, his mother, nor her friend were ever together during ministry. Dee Dee and Dawnetta's first priority was to ascertain that Grady was born again, which he was. They assessed him to be very spiritually weak as a Christian, and discovered that he had never been baptized in the Holy Spirit. They taught him about the baptism in the Holy Spirit, and then prayed for him. He received that infilling and began praying in his prayer language. Above all, he convinced them of his deep desire to be well.

They had to give him frequent breaks because Grady's attention span was about fifteen to twenty minutes - maximum. In addition, he was heavily medicated and slept a great deal. He also interacted with the voices in his head almost constantly. He believed that a cop had implanted a microchip in his brain.

Unlike the way most schizophrenics are treated, we never tried to convince Grady that the voices in his head didn't exist. In fact, we believed that they did exist. Our team's biggest challenge was convincing Grady that these entities were not his friends, and that God's power was greater than theirs.

We used our authority to bind, muzzle and gag the spirits, and although they never manifested themselves to us, they spoke to Grady continually trying to sabotage the process. It was important for us to know what they were telling him. When a stronghold was about to be broken, Grady would get very agitated and demanding. *"I have to go to the bathroom! I have to go to the bathroom! I have to go to the bathroom right now!"*

We could hear his side of the conversation from the bathroom. *"I know! I know!"* he said. *"I'll just pretend. It's all right! We'll make sure they think that."*

Grady came out of the bathroom and said, *"Okay…they're gone. We're done. They're dead."*

Each time, we would redirect him back to the reality that they weren't gone and help him choose again to be free. *"Grady, can you see that Michelle is not your friend? She is making your life miserable."*

Grady's maturation level was very young so we spoke simply and used hand gestures when we spoke. When he was carrying on a conversation with the demons we said slowly, *"Stop! We're not listening to that! We're going to trust God!"* We acted out each sentence.

Eventually when the voices spoke to him, Grady would say with hand gestures, *"Stop! We're not listening to that! We're going to trust God!"*

After fifteen or twenty minutes Grady would be ready for a break. As soon as we stopped working, he would fall asleep. While he slept, we prayed the healing prayers for schizophrenia over him. We did this repeatedly so that the prayers would be imprinted on his spirit.

As a starting place for the deliverance, we used the list of spiritual strongholds for schizophrenia listed in the book *Pigs in a Parlour* by Frank and Ida Mae Hammond. In this book, Hammond portrays schizophrenia as two hands, one with the stronghold of rejection and the other with a stronghold of rebellion. Each hand lists the demonic branches that stem from those two roots, with paranoia as a type of handcuff that ties to two hands together.

We began by dealing with rejection. When we'd finished with that, we were left with one angry, rebellious teen. In working with children and teens, we always try to keep the experience pleasant so that they never want to run from God or His people. However, as anger erupted in Grady, we had to put up the same firm boundaries that we do with our own teens.

"I'm done!" he'd say. *"I don't want to do this!"*

"Sit down," we'd say. *"Now...this is what we need to do. We need you to tell us if you really want to get free and be well. It's your choice."*

He really did want to be free so he'd settle down and get back to work until the demons got him agitated again.

"Excuse me! Stop listening to that demon. That behavior is not acceptable." We also made a point to pour in God's virtue in every place where something was removed from him.

In addition to the spirits listed in *Pigs in a Parlor,* we listened to Grady to find out what other specific things needed to be dealt with. For instance, a few of the demonic entities we dealt with were the microchip, the cop, Michael and Michelle.

At first we did all the warfare on his behalf, but as Grady got stronger, we put a demand on him. *"No, you make him stop talking."*

Eventually we could hear him in the bathroom saying, *"Shut up in Jesus' name! I don't want you!"* As he took more control over the demons, his attention span improved. We prayed prayers to heal the trauma in his life, and we also prayed that God would bring him quickly up to his chronological and maturational age.

By the end of our sessions on the second day, we knew we'd done all we could for Grady at that time. There was no way his life would ever be the same, but we weren't jumping up and down with joy because we knew Michelle wasn't gone. This demon had convinced Grady that she was his friend, and Grady was lonely enough that he wasn't ready to give her up. *"You're ultimately going to have to say goodbye to Michelle,"* we told him. But in the meantime, we just had to trust God.

After Care

On the third day the team taught Grady, his mother and her friend what it would take to keep his deliverance. The key points that we taught his mother were as follows:

- You cannot ask for change and accept old behavior
- You have to make a shift in your mind and treat him differently

- Don't accept his talking to demons
- If it happens a hundred times a day, deal with it a hundred times a day
- Expect him to act like a healed person acts
- Treat him as though he were a normal young man even if he isn't acting like one yet
- Pray over him and over his room daily
- Plead the blood of Jesus over his mind even while he sleeps
- Pray the 91st Psalm over him daily

Grady's mother was extremely motivated to see him set free and healed. We told her that the healing process would take time. Until now it had been okay for him to interact out loud with the demons and ignore everyone in the room, but it was no longer okay, so the whole family would have to relate to him in a different manner.

The main things we taught Grady were as follows:

- You have to trust God to help you find your identity in Christ Jesus
- Read the Bible like you've never read it before
- Pray in your prayer language daily
- Play praise and worship music
- Never speak to demons unless it is to make them leave
- They will come back and lie to you. Don't believe them!
- Don't watch television, movies, or listen to music that doesn't glorify God
- Spend time each day listening to the Holy Spirit
- Put on the full armor of God daily
- Focus on Jesus

The last day we spent together was fun, and they attended church with us that night. Grady sat through the entire service without a problem. Afterwards, he went to dinner with a large group, including other teens, none of whom ever suspected that he had a problem.

The First Year

Grady's family saw an immediate improvement. They watched as God brought Grady through developmental stages that he'd missed as a child. *"One day he'd be picking his nose like a three year old,"* his mother wrote. *"Another day he'd be wrestling with his brothers like a ten year old. The next thing I knew he was asking for his driver's permit!"*

When Grady returned home to finish summer school with his tutor, the Special Education Supervisor for the high school he would be attending, she noticed Grady's improvement immediately. Grady had improved so much that instead of putting him back in a private room for three hours of one-on-one education as they'd planned, she recommended that he have five hours a day of remedial classes with a para-professional at his side.

Two days after school started, she called to brag about how well Grady was doing. Two days later Grady's mother got a second call. *"We'll have to make some changes,"* she was told. Her heart sank.

"Grady is bored in remedial physical education and wants to be in regular physical education." These weren't the kind of reports that she was used to hearing!

Ninth grade went smoothly, and Grady handled his classes so well that two more classes were added to his schedule.

Follow-Up Ministry

In July of 2003, Grady's mother brought him back to Oklahoma for a follow-up deliverance. The first thing the team noticed about Grady was the change in his attention span. Instead of working for fifteen minutes at a stretch, he could stay engaged for four hours. The previous lying and manipulative behavior was absent, and he seemed much more at peace.

Over the past year Grady had a taste of freedom. He'd been able to see and experience a level of freedom he hadn't known was possible. He'd made some poor choices that led him into pornography. He'd also made a poor choice to listen to music by the Insane Clown Posse, which had reinforced a spirit of insanity. Now in addition to Michelle, he had been joined by Rebecca, a gang spirit that kept him mentally "protected." They'd also been joined by Jessica, a third demonic entity.

"Michelle doesn't like you because you take her power away," Grady explained.

He was learning that she wasn't all powerful!

Now that he'd had a taste of freedom, Grady was ready to get rid of everything that stood in his way. But Michelle played on his emotions.

Dawnetta had a particular understanding of the power a "friend" can have over a lonely person. Due to a trauma that happened in her life at age two, rejection became her "friend." It lied to her making her believe it was protecting her. It wasn't until she was an adult that she was faced with the realization that she had to chose between God and this childhood chum. It was the hardest decision she'd ever made, and she grieved over the loss of a friend, even a bad one. She relayed the story to Grady.

"Michelle says that she loves me and will take care of me."

"You know that's a lie. She has never taken care of you."

"I can hear her crying!" Grady said.

"I'm sorry, but that is a demon who is manipulating your emotions. Emotions lie and you can't be led by them."

"But..."

"You've got a choice to make, Grady. What are you going to do?"

"Goodbye, Michelle," he said, *"you have to go."*

This time when Grady flew home, he did not take any excess baggage.

Progress Report

In August of 2003, Grady started tenth grade with a para-professional in each class. Within two weeks she was dismissed from his physical education and art classes. Later she removed herself from his history class. Because he still struggled with math and science, she continued to help him with those subjects. As Grady improved over the past two years, his doctor gradually weaned him off the medication until he was taking only a fraction of what he'd previously taken.

By the summer of 2004, he had attended Bible Camp and held down two jobs. Grady is a currently a junior in high school where he attends some remedial classes and some mainstream classes. Already this year, teachers have commented on the improved alertness and greater, though not complete, independence that Grady is showing.

Jesus is still in the business of setting the captives free.

He who the Son set's free - is free indeed.

Publishers' Note: In May 2006, I stayed with Pat and Dee in Oklahoma City. Grady had recently graduated from high School in the previous month. This is a real miracle!

Chapter Three

Genetics and Generational Iniquity

"So God created man in his own image, in the image of God created he him; male and female created he them." Genesis 1:27

"And God saw every thing that he had made, and, behold, it was very good. And the evening and the morning were the sixth day." Genesis 1:31

If God said it was very good, it was very good. I believe that at the time of creation every gene, every chromosome, every part of the genome interacted perfectly. When man sinned, the door was opened allowing damage to God's perfect creation.. When you consider the intricacies of the human body with 30,000 genes and 3 million base pairs, it is amazing that our bodies still function as well as they do with all the possibilities of damage. Just think of the imperfections that we take for granted, near-sighted, balding, greying of the hair, these are all part of the damage that iniquity has done to the genes. I understand that there are many diseases and malfunctions of the body caused by bacteria, viruses, accidents etc. not related to gene damage. What I want to cover in this book is related to the genes and how damage to them causes problems.

In 2004 at the conference, *Clash of the Kingdoms*, Ana Mendez taught on iniquities. Her teaching rocked my theology when she said iniquity was passed down through the spirit. Prayerfully seeking God's instruction, it began to make sense to me. If God knew us before the foundation of the earth, we had to have been spirit. If iniquity is passed down to the 3rd and 4th generations, (Exodus 30:5) the DNA must start in the spirit. So the spiritual DNA must affect the physical DNA.

"His disciples asked Him, Rabbi, who sinned, this man or his parents, that he should be born blind? Jesus answered, It was not that this man or his parents sinned, but he was born blind in order that the workings of God should be manifested (displayed and illustrated) in him." (John 9:2-3 AMP)

Jesus didn't seem surprised that they asked this question. In Jesus' day it was common knowledge that sin caused physical problems. Another Scripture that supports this is Mark 2:5

"When Jesus saw their faith, he said to the paralytic, "Son, your sins are forgiven." (NIV)

In Henry Wright's book, *A More Excellent Way,* Pleasant Valley Publications 1999, he observes a number of diseases and their root causes. This is not a scientific study, however it is a good starting point. I believe we must seek God on each case and ask what generational iniquity is present.

It is helpful to know the exact iniquity producing the disorder, allowing our prayers to be specific. This is not always possible. When the specific iniquity is not known, we need to repent for any sin in our generations that may have caused iniquities resulting in genetic damage.

The field of genetics is moving so fast it's incredible. Preparing to speak in Dallas in July, 2005 I was looking for examples of disease processes that would clearly show how sin can damage a gene. I thought of lung cancer. Pollutants in the air, especially cigarette smoke are the #1 cause of this disease. I looked up the genetics of lung cancer in May and found that only one cell type, of the four I was familiar with, had a genetic connection. I looked it up again in October 2005 to write a prayer. Then, only five months later, 49 genes believed to be related to lung cancer were listed.

Of these 49 damaged genes, many are not inherited but are initiated in that individual. The damage to the genes is caused by pollutants in the air, the most common being cigarette smoke. The obvious sin to be repented for is the sin of our nation not taking care of the atmosphere. We must repent for our own sin of smoking and forgive others for smoking and exposing us to second hand smoke. The damage the pollutant does occurs at the genetic level and science has not discovered a treatment for this level of damage. We can treat damage at the cellular level. Stem cell research is science's attempt to treat disease at the genetic level.

When you look at the root causes of diseases listed in Henry Wright's book you will see fear, anger, bitterness, self hatred, etc. You may wonder how these emotions could cause damage to the genes. When you experience any of these emotions, your body produces a chemical reaction in an attempt to maintain balance. When you have a prolonged episode of one or more of these emotions, thc chemical reaction can cause damagc. Stress leading to hypertension and worry leading to ulcers would be examples.

Chapter Four

A Study of Genetics

It took a lot of time and patience for Dee to bring me up to a level of understanding so I could teach on the topic of genetics. While this is in no way intended to be a medical journal, I would like to give you a simple overview of how the genes and chromosomes are related and how damage can affect a person. We will start with some definitions.

Iniquity *– An iniquity, according to Strong's 5753, is to make crooked, pervert, or do wickedly. So when a sin, which is missing the mark is committed, it can begin an iniquitous pattern that damages a gene which is then passed down generationally.*

The Human Genome Project *– A study of the entire genetic system began in 1990. In 2003 a draft of the entire human genome was completed. Although many of the genes, and all of the chromosomes have been identified, we are in the infantile stages of mapping disease processes. I am in no way intending to give a detailed teaching on the genome system, but I would like to give you some facts and analogies that will help you understand where and how damage at this level works so you will be able to pray effectively for its healing.*

Imagine the human genome as a library. A chromosome is a book in the library. There is no one theme for each chromosome. There are varying numbers of bands on each chromosome, they are the chapters in the book. A gene is a sentence in the chapter. There are 30,000 genes. There are thousands of genes on each chromosome. Each gene or sentence gives directions for cell function. For instance, some genes tell the bone marrow how to produce blood cells. Another group of genes tells the eye how to constrict when too much light comes in. Some genes tell the hair what texture it is to be while some are in charge of eye colour, skin color, hair color and whether the hair is curly or straight.

Base pairs are the letters that make up the words of the sentences. Each person has 3,000,000,000 base pairs, this is equal to 200 volumes of 1,000 page telephone books. If you change one letter in a word, you will change the whole meaning of a sentence. So if there is a sin that affects the base pair, it will then affect the gene. There are actually only 4 letters in the genetic code, A,T,C and G, but for our purposes we will use the English alphabet for demonstration.

The Beginning of Life. When the sperm and ovum are joined, each parent gives 23 chromosomes. These chromosomes are given randomly. The father may give 10 of the chromosomes he received from his father and 13 he received from his mother. The mother may give 8 she received from her father and 15 she received from her mother. I asked a math teacher to figure out the combinations that were possible from this random match. The figure he got was 70 trillion, 38 billion, 744 million, 177 thousand 664 different possibilities from this 23 chromosome mix. This is just from these two generations. This is the reason we are all different. This is also the reason diseases aren't always inherited. If your mother has a gene from her father for diabetes and one from her mother that is healthy, and she passes the healthy one to you, you will not have the propensity for diabetes, unless your father passes you a gene that has that damage.

"I will praise You; for I am fearfully and wonderfully made: marvellous are they works; and that my soul knows very well." (Psalm 139:14)

The Human Genome - The Library

In humans, each cell normally contains 23 pairs of chromosomes, for a total of 46. Twenty-two of these pairs, called autosomes, look the same in both males and females. The 23rd pair, the sex chromosomes, differ between males and females. Females have two copies of the X chromosome, while males have one X and one Y chromosome.

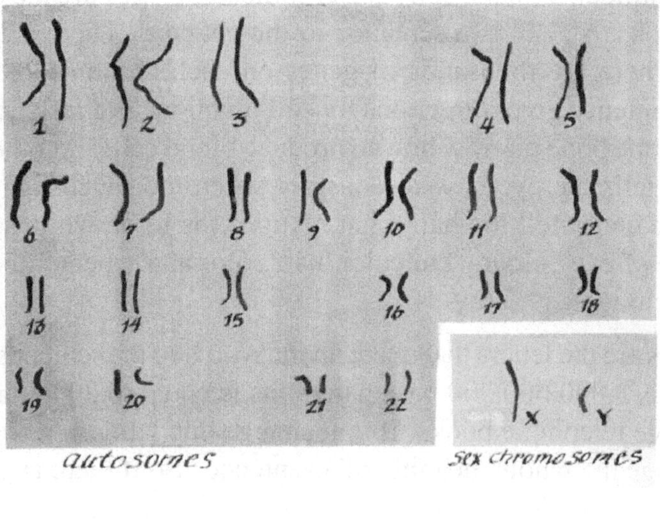

Each chromosome pairs with the corresponding chromosome. Chromosome 1 with chromosome 1 etc. They are numbered from the largest to the smallest. The location of the genes on the chromosomes also correspond.

CHROMOSOMES BEFORE THEY JOIN AS PAIRS

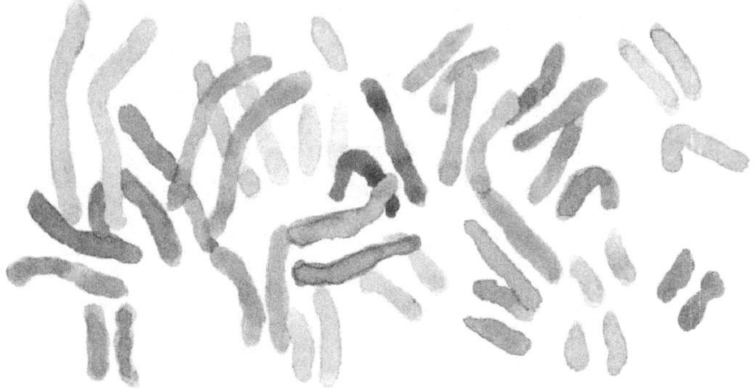

As you can see, they have all found their partners except the sex chromosomes as represented by the single pale blue and the single pink chromosome.

CHROMOSOMAL LOCATION OF A GENE

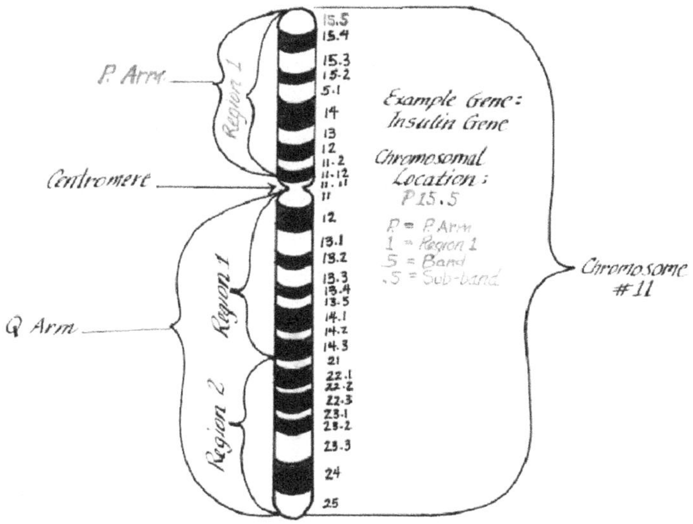

This is a picture of chromosome 11. The bands that you see are the chapters, or location of the genes. Each chromosome is divided by an indention called the centromere. The chromosome has a short arm and a long arm. If the gene is found on the short arm, its location begins with p and the number indicates the distance from the centromere. The smaller the number the closer to the centromere. If the gene is on the long arm its location begins with q followed by a number, again indicating the distance from the centromere. This picture shows chromosome 11 with the insulin gene located at region 1; on band 5 and sub-band 5 of the short arm. Therefore its address is 11 (for the chromosome) p because it's the short arm 15.5. It would look like this, Gene, the Insulin Gene, chromosomal location 11p15.5.

Chromosome Pair

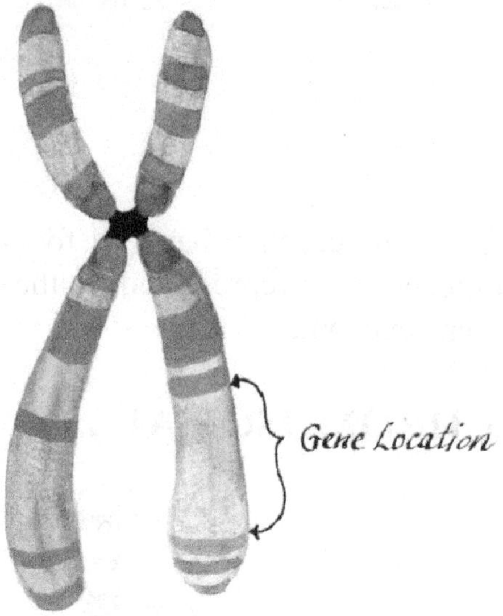

The chromosome from the mother and the chromosome from the father join at the centromere. This picture shows the two joined with the bands indicating where genes are located.

Chromosome Pairs with Corresponding Genes

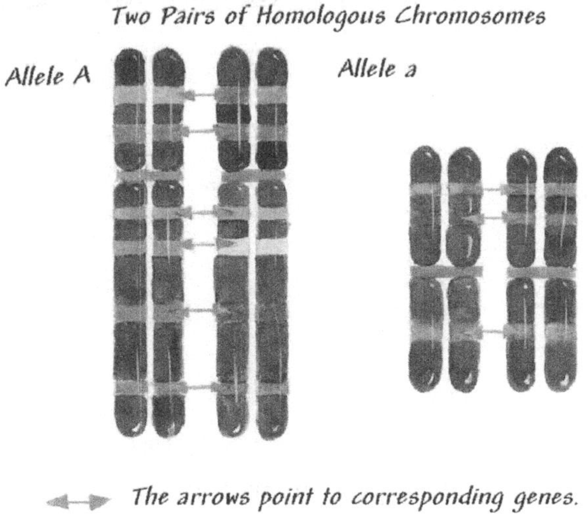

This picture shows the pairs with the genes that match. Sometimes the genes are exactly the same, but if we are dealing with different expressions of the same function like the texture of hair if one is for straight hair and one for curly, the genes appear a little different as indicated by a different color. This is the way all the chromosomes pair up except the sex chromosomes. Since the X chromosome is much bigger than the Y chromosome, most of the genes on the X chromosome do not have corresponding genes on the Y chromosome.

Genes are made up of DNA.
Each chromosome contains many genes.

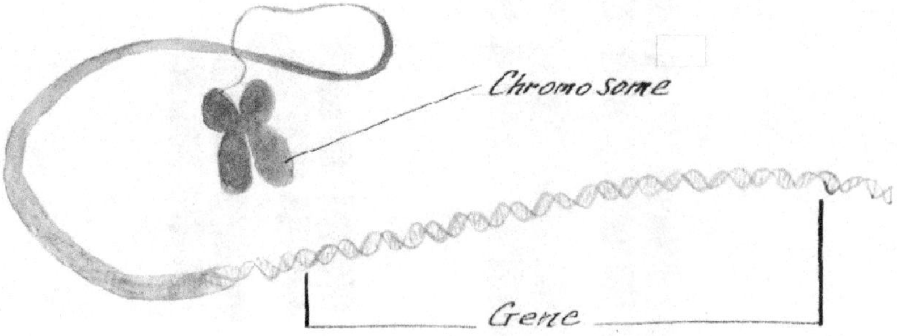

The genes are tightly wrapped in protein and attached to the chromosomes on the different bands inside the chromosomes

DNA is a double helix formed by base pairs attached to a sugar-phosphate backbone.

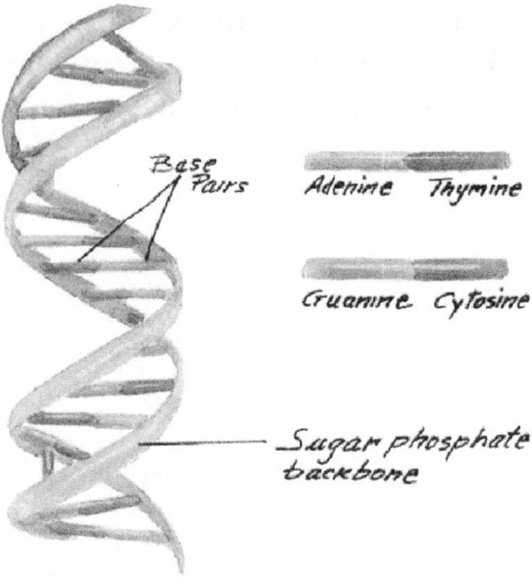

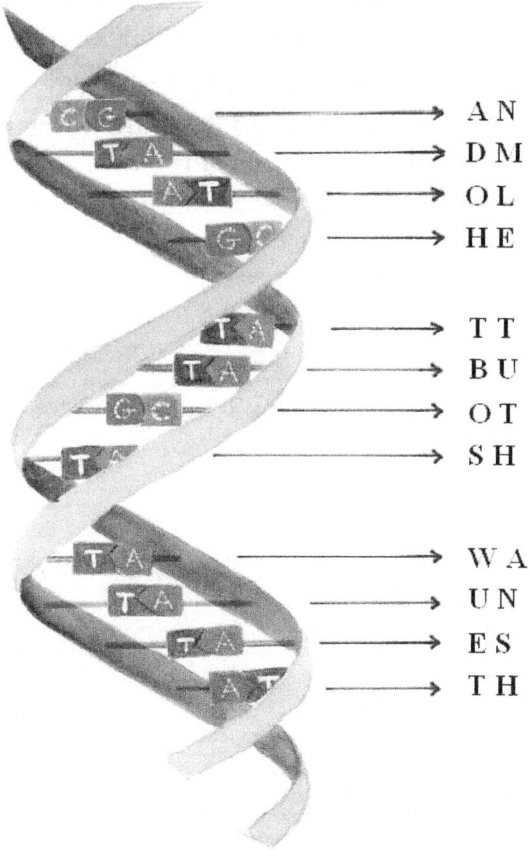

It's the sequencing or order of the base pairs that determines the gene's instructions to the cells. On the actual DNA strand you can see the 4 letters that actually make up the base pairs. Outside of the picture you can see our sentence starting at the bottom, "The sun was hot but the old man……."

We can think about the DNA sequence of a gene as a sentence made up entirely of three – letter words. "Thesunwashotbuttheoldmandidnotgethishat."

If you split these letter into individual three-letter words, it would read, **"The sun was hot but the old man did not get his hat."** This would be a healthy gene. But if you shifted the three – letter reading frame one letter it would read, "t hew unw ash otb utt heo ldm and idn otg eth ish at," or th esu nwa sho tbu tth eol dma ndi dno tge thi sha t. Only one of these reading frames translates into an understandable sentence. In the same way, only one three – letter reading frame within a gene codes for the correct protein (instruction to the cell.)

Let's look at Schizophrenia. One of the chromosomes affected in Schizophrenia if Chromosome 22.

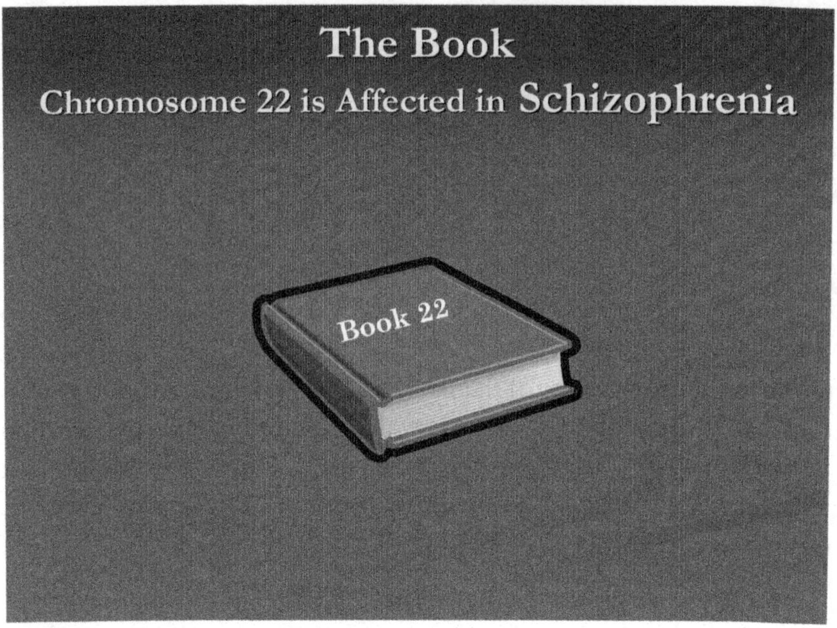

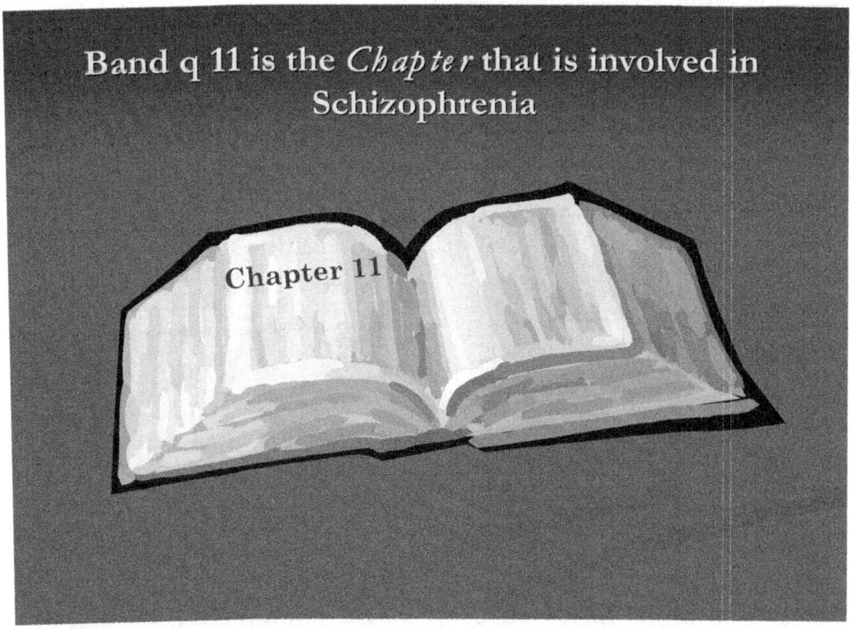

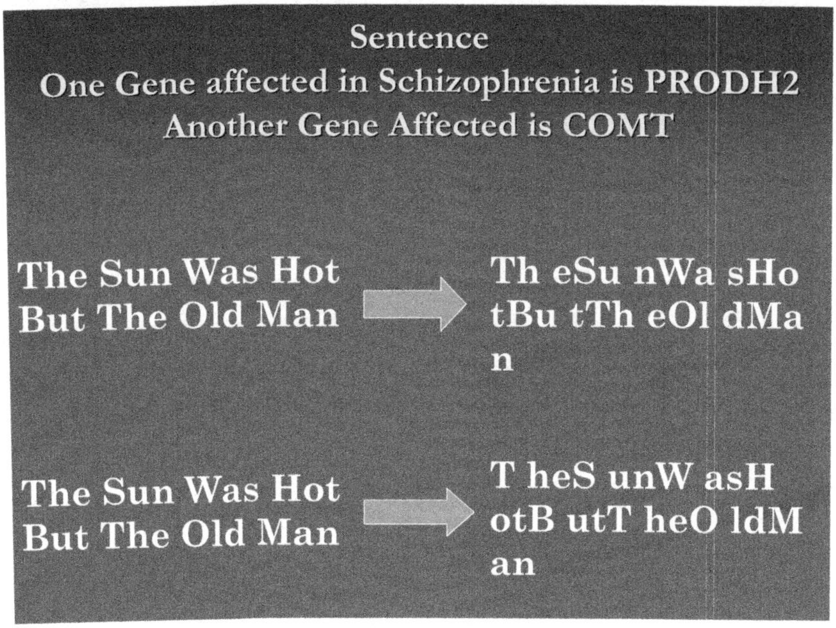

A gene damaged by sin will be passed down generationally in the damaged or mutated form.

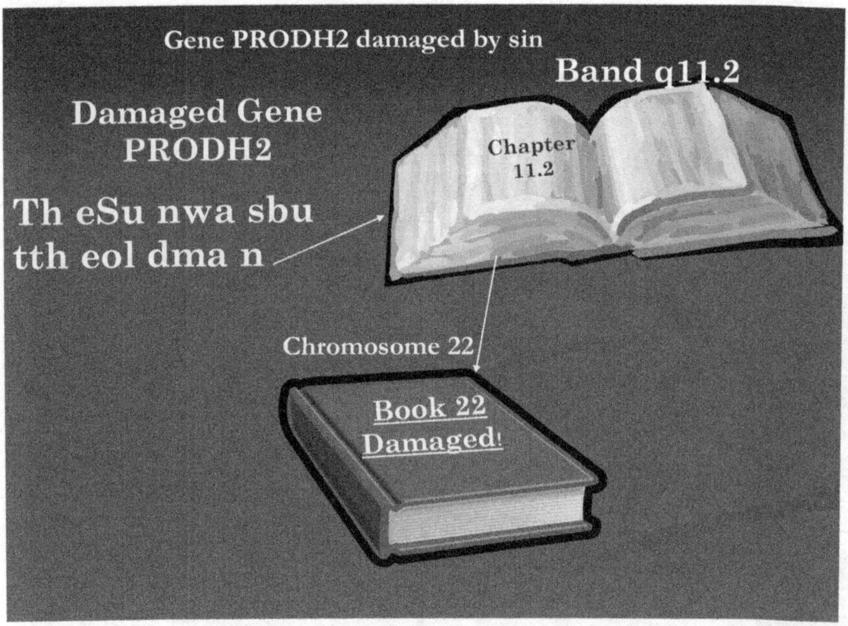

Here is what it looks like. Gene PRODH2 is damaged. It is passed down in a damaged state. It is located on band q11. 2. Band q11.2 is a chapter or location in Chromosome 22. So now there is damage to the chromosome. Now that person has a propensity for schizophrenia. A stress occurs in his life and the schizophrenia manifests. Henry Wright states in his book *A More Excellent Way* that schizophrenia is not a genetic based disease. His observation is that schizophrenia is based in fear and there is a chemical imbalance involved. We must remember that he first published his book in 1999. The first draft of the human Genome project was in 2003. I don't know when scientists discovered the genetic mutation that causes schizophrenia, but most of us old timers in medicine would tell you we were taught it was not a genetic-based disease.

Most schizophrenia manifests in a person's life in his 20s. Either when he leaves the security of his home and goes to college, or embarks on a career. The stress causes the chemical imbalance that Henry Wright describes, but the propensity for the disease is already there and manifests. Gene COMT is also thought to be associated with schizophrenia. It is also located on chromosome 22 band q11.21. We have included both genes in the prayer we have written for healing of schizophrenia.

As I was praying about a way to explain this, the Lord gave me another analogy. When I was nine years old we moved to a house that was a fixer-upper. My dad was a carpenter and for the next few years we were in a constant state of remodeling. He built the kitchen as an add on from the ground up. This house had a conventional foundation set on concrete blocks with joists and a sub floor. My sister and I were ages 8 and 10 when we were given the job of nailing the sub-floor to the joists. We would race to the end of our board bending half of the nails as we went. About two years later while sitting at the kitchen table it hit me that we hadn't finished nailing the sub-floor! I could imagine the floor shifting and buckling under our weight and movement because it wasn't secure. I told my dad and he laughed and assured me that he had completed what we had missed. What the Lord showed me is this. When a gene is not connected to the chromosome properly, stress can cause it to slip or buckle and the manifestation of the disease will occur. It will depend on how many "nails" were left out and how much stress is applied. If the board (gene) is just lying in place on the joist (chromosome), but not attached at all, it will take less stress. Another possibility is that the board is rotten (or the gene is so damaged) that no amount of nails will hold it. In this instance, it would not take much stress for the board to break and the floor to sink.

Chapter Five
A Brief Look at Diabetes

Many chromosomes are involved in diabetes. Some are involved in type 1 diabetes and some are involved in type 2 diabetes. Chromosomes 2,5,6,10,11,14 and 18 are involved in Type 1 Diabetes. Chromosomes 2,3,11,17 and 20 are involved in Type 2 Diabetes.

Chromosomes 2, 5, 6, 10, 11, 14, and 18 are Involved with Type 1 Diabetes

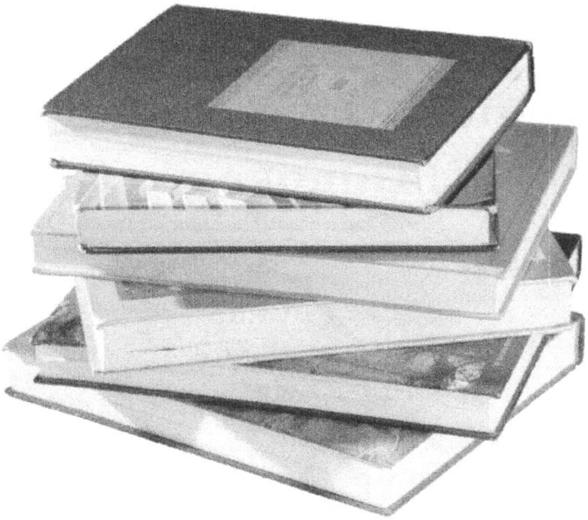

The different genes involved that are attached to these chromosomes are implicated with different aspects of glucose formation, metabolism and utilization.

Two genes are major culprits in causing diabetes. DQB 1 and DRB 1. In the making of Gene DQB 1 the sequencing or letters in the base pairs are affected making the meaning of the words different thus the gene is not formed properly.

Damage to Gene DQB 1

DQB1

The sun was hot but the old man did not get his hat.

Th esu nwa sho tbu tth eol dma ndi dno tge thi sha t.

This gene is now mutated and has a different expression, it now produces the wrong amino acid.

Gene DQB 1 Damages Chromosome 6

Gene DQB1

1. **Th esu nwa sho tbu tth eol dma ndi dno tge thi sha t.**

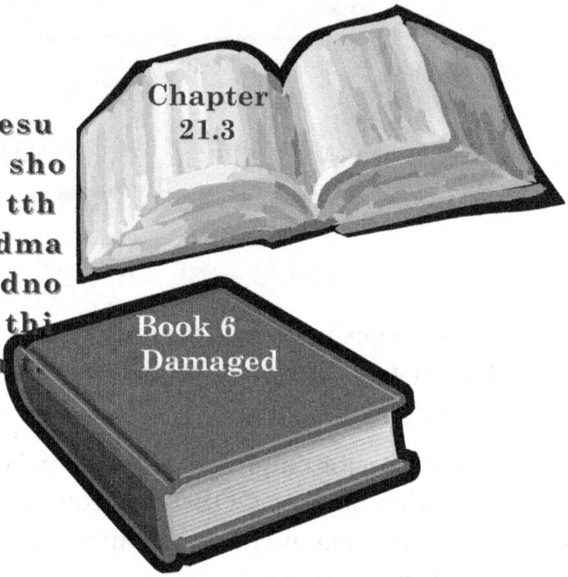

Whether we use the analogy of the letters not making sense or the board not being nailed down properly, the gene is not attached to the chromosome properly. This chromosome is now damaged.

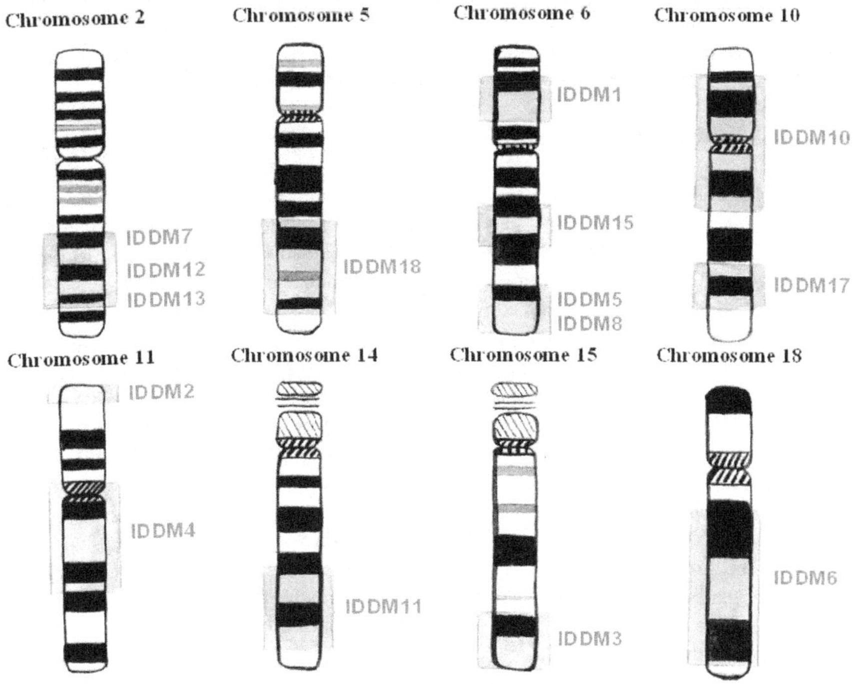

Several chromosomes are involved in diabetes. This shows each chromosome with the bands or the chapters where the genes are located. We have these chromosomes with the specific genes in each region in the prayer for the healing of diabetes.

The Insulin Gene

This gene has 2200 base pairs. This is a good example of part of the gene expressing itself properly and part of it scrambled. This gene is located on chromosome 11p15.5 and affects both type 1 and type 2 diabetes. The following is an example of what 2200 base pairs look like when some are in the right order and some are scrambled.

* The sun was hot but the old man did not get his hat. T hes unw ash otb utt heo ldm and idn otg eth ish at. The sun was hot but the old man did not get his hat. The sun was hot but the old man did not get his hat. T hes unw ash otb utt heo ldm and idn otg eth ish at. The sun was hot but the old man did not get his hat. The sun was hot but the old man did not get his hat. T hes unw ash otb utt heo ldm and idn otg eth ish at. The sun was hot but the old man did not get his hat. The sun was hot but the old man did not get his hat. T hes unw ash otb utt heo ldm and idn otg eth ish at. The sun was hot but the old man did not get his hat.The sun was hot but the old man did not get his hat. T hes unw ash otb utt heo ldm and idn otg eth ish at. The sun was hot but the old man did not get his hat. The sun was hot but the old man did not get his hat. T hes unw ash otb utt heo ldm and idn otg eth ish at. The sun was hot but the old man did not get his hat. The sun was hot but the old man did not get his hat. T hes unw ash otb utt heo ldm and idn otg eth ish at. The sun was hot but the old man did not get his hat. The sun was hot but the old man did not get his hat. T hes unw ash otb utt heo ldm and idn otg eth ish at. The sun was hot but the old man did not get his hat. The sun was hot but the old man did not get his hat. T hes unw ash otb utt heo ldm and idn otg eth ish at. The sun was hot but the old man did not get his hat. The sun was hot but the old man did not get his hat. T hes unw ash otb utt heo ldm and idn otg eth ish at. The sun was hot but the old man did not get his hat. The sun was hot but the old man did not get his hat. T hes unw ash otb utt heo ldm and idn otg eth ish at. The sun was hot but the old man did not get his hat. The sun was hot but the old man did not get his hat. T hes unw ash otb utt heo ldm and idn otg eth ish at. The sun was hot but the old man did not get his hat. The sun was hot but the old man did not get his hat. T hes unw ash otb utt heo ldm and idn otg eth ish at. The sun was hot but the old man did not get his hat. The sun was hot but the old man did not get his hat. T hes unw ash otb utt heo ldm and idn otg eth ish at. The sun was hot but the old man did not get his hat. The sun was hot but the old man did not get his hat. T hes unw ash otb utt heo ldm and idn otg eth ish at. The sun was hot but the old man did not get his hat. The sun was hot but the old man did not get his hat. T hes unw ash otb utt heo ldm and idn otg eth ish at. The sun was hot but the old man did not get his hat. The sun was hot but the old man did not get his hat. T hes unw ash otb utt heo ldm and idn otg eth ish at. The sun was hot but the old man did not get his hat. The sun was hot but the old man did not get his hat. T hes unw ash otb utt heo ldm and idn otg eth ish at. The sun was hot but the old man did not get his hat. The sun was hot but the old man did not get his hat. T hes unw ash otb utt heo ldm and idn otg eth ish at. The sun was hot but the old man did not get his hat. The sun was hot but the o

With this gene involved, the person has a propensity for both Type 1 and Type 2 Diabetes.

Chapter Six

How to Write a Prayer for a Genetic-Based Disorder

I have included several prayers in chapter seven of this book. We start each prayer with repenting because of the sins of our forefathers which caused an iniquitous pattern to be passed down through our generations. We then forgive our ancestors for passing that iniquitous pattern down and for any damage it did to cause a genetic based disorder. I recommend Henry Wright's book, *A More Excellent Way*, as a place to start to identify any possible sin for which to repent.

Next we pray for healing of any physical damage in our body. This part of the prayer may be short or it may be lengthy depending on the physical condition of the person being prayed for. For instance, when praying for diabetes we pray that God would heal and restore the cardiovascular system, the eyes, the kidneys, the nerves and other organ system or cells that have been damaged by diabetes. We pray that God heal the pancreas and cause it to function properly.

After that we pray for the genome system. To find the genes and chromosomes that are affected in a particular disorder we did the following. Go on line and type into your search engine the name of the disease and genetics, i.e. "schizophrenia genetics." I will warn you that many sites will be available and it takes time to visit each site to see if there is information concerning a specific gene and its location. Some of the research is animal based but I used only the results found in humans. There is a lot to evaluate but after you get used to spotting the addresses, i.e. chromosome 22q11 or chromosome 7p3.2-3.5, you will be able to skim over the rest. When you see an address like the last example, it simple means that there are genes along that chromosome from the area 3.2-3.5. Looking at the examples of the prayers we have written you will see that often the name of the gene is known but sometimes you will only know the location. Pray as specifically as possible. If you have the name of the gene, use it, if not, pray for the healing of the genes on the location listed.

Two web-sites that were very helpful to me in understanding the Human Genome System were, **"The Human_Genome/launchpad and The Genetic Science Learning Center: (http://www.ornl.gov/sci/techresources/Human_Genome/launchpad/)** and, **"The Genetic Science Learning Center: The Basics and Beyond" (http://gslc.genetics.utah.edu/).**

Chapter Seven
Prayers

Healing Prayer for Schizophrenia

1. Have the person repent because of the sins of his ancestors especially the sin of fear that allowed an iniquitous pattern to be passed down through his generations. Have him forgive his ancestors for passing that iniquitous pattern down and for any damage it did to cause a genetic based disorder. Have him repent for his own sins as well.

2. Pray that God will heal any structural brain abnormalities and any defects on the human genome that may have been passed down through the generations or were caused by a virus, stress, or other factors.

3. Pray specifically for Chromosome 22Q11 that any genes that are attached to that chromosome will be healed and properly aligned.

4. Pray for the healing of chromosomes 2, 10 and 22. Pray that the Lord would heal any translocations especially involving chromosomes 10P11-15 to 22Q12 in the DNA structure of the individual.

5. Pray that God will restore any gene that has mutated back to the structure that He planned for it to be from the foundation of the earth. Pray that any mutated gene be healed and restored whether it was passed down in a mutated state or has suffered mutation from a virus or any other reason.

6. Pray that God will properly align any genes that are not lined up as they should be on the chromosomes.

7. Ask God to heal any changes in these genes or how they attach to the chromosomes.

8. Ask God to heal any mutations located on chromosomes 7q11, 8p21-p22, 14q13,

9. Pray for the specific genes PRODH2 and COMT that are located on chromosome 22q11.2. Ask that any changes or deletions in the makeup of their protein that causes an inborn error of metabolism

that would cause schizophrenia be healed and restored to what God intended for it to be.

10. Ask God to cause any enzyme that is associated with, produced by, or controlled by PRODH2 or COMT to be balanced and brought into alignment with His original plan.

11. Ask God to cause any deletions, abnormalities or lack of COMT that may be caused by a gene mutation to be healed and restored. If needed, Lord create, adjust, and/or restore this gene. We pray that whether it is passed down in a mutated state or if it suffered mutation within this, that you would heal or recreate it. Ask God to heal and restore each base pair to its intended function.

12. Pray that God would heal gene DISC 2 on chromosome 1q42.1.

13. Pray that God would heal gene DTNBP1 on chromosome 6p22.3.

14. Pray that God would heal gene GRM3 on chromosome 7q21.12.

15. Pray that God would heal gene NRG1 on chromosome 8.

16. Pray that God would heal gene SCZD7 on chromosome 13q32.

17. Pray that God would heal gene CHRNA7 on chromosome 15q14.

18. Pray that God would heal genes APP, AAA, CVAP and AD1 on chromosome 21q21.

19. Pray that God would heal gene DBCR6 on chromosome 22.

20. Pray healing to the neurotransmitters, receptors and synapse.

21. Pray that God would balance the amount of dopamine and serotonin to create levels that would bring normal healthy and healed function.

22. Pray that the brain chemicals would allow the Godly communication between each brain cell to receive and retrieve information normally. Pray that the total healing of the synapse, axiom and synaptic fluid would be balanced to act and react according to God's original plan for them to function.

23. Pray that the Lord would heal the cortical structure in the midsection of the brain's lobes.

24. Pray that the Lord would heal the pre-frontal cortex and lobular areas.

25. Pray that the Lord would synchronize the neurotransmitters that are producing nor-epinephrine, dopamine and serotonin, regulating them to interact in a way that will cause healing and health.

26. Pray that the Lord would remove any pathway and brain wiring that is looped and destructive.

27. Pray that the Lord would release His power to heal and create as well as redesign any and all pathways in the brain that need His healing touch.

28. Thank God for restoring function of the genes and chromosomes we have listed.

29. Thank God for healing and restoring the function of the genes and chromosomes involved in schizophrenia that we don't know about. We thank you God that You are our creator, know us intimately and You know each and every defect down to the base pair of our genome structure that needs restoration.

AMEN

Prayer for Bipolar Disorder

1. Pray that God will heal any structural brain abnormalities that have been passed down through the generations.

2. Pray that God will heal any changes of some of the linkages or disturbances in make-up or placement of genes.

3. Pray that God will restore any gene that has mutated to the structure as He planned for it to be from the foundation of the earth. Pray that any mutated gene be healed and restored whether it was passed down in a mutated state or has suffered mutation from any other reason, whether it be from the effects of drugs or manic or depressive episodes.

4. Come against any generational curse or sin that caused the mutation of a gene or genes that have been passed down.

5. Pray that God will properly align any genes that are not lined up as they should be on the chromosomes.

6. Ask God to heal any changes in these genes or how they attach to the chromosomes and heal the expression of the way the proteins are expressed within the genes.

7. Ask God to heal and restore each base pair to its intended function.

8. Pray that God will heal the electrical firing system of the components of the brain whether to slow down the excessive firing or fill in the skips and restore it to the way He intended before the foundation of the earth.

Prayer for ADD and ADHD

1. Lord I pray that You would heal this one of any structural brain abnormalities that have been passed down through the generations or that have been caused by stress in the womb.

2. Lord I pray that You would heal the transmitters, axiom and synapse within this one's brain function to normalize the firing and receptors to be normal. I pray that the amino acids and chemical releases would normalize and neutrons would perform and function normally.

3. Ask God to heal and restore each base pair to its intended function.

4. Lord I pray that You would adjust and heal those parts of the brain that need healing especially in these parts according to this individuals needs:

- In the cerebral cortex, prefrontal and frontal lobe.
- In the parietal lobe and the occipital lobes
- In the temporal lobes and the brain stem.
- In the cerebellum.
- In the thalamus and the hypothalamus areas.
- In the Broca's Aphasia and the Wernecke's area.

5. Lord I pray for the neurological interruptions and over firing to normalize. I ask You to balance and renew the neurological pathways and brain wiring to be routed in a way that would bring health and healing to this person.

6. I bind the familiar spirits of ADD and ADHD.

7. I bind the spirits of rejection, self-hatred, rebellion, jealousy and envy.

8. I bind the Deaf and Dumb spirits and any Beelzebub babbling spirit.

9. I bind any homosexual spirits and double-minded spirits in the name of Jesus.

10. I pray for a release of your healing power in the name of Jesus.

Healing Prayer for Diabetes

1. Have the person repent because of the sins of his ancestors especially the sin of self-hatred, self rejection, guilt, fear and anxiety that allowed an iniquitous pattern to be passed down through his generations. Have him forgive his ancestors for passing that iniquitous pattern down and for any damage it did to cause a genetic based disorder. Have him repent for his own sins as well.

2. Pray that God would heal any defects leading to the predisposition, development, manifestation and continuation of diabetes mellitus.

3. Pray that God would heal any defects of the genome of this individual.

4. Pray that God would heal every defect of this individuals chromosomes. Pray specifically for healing of chromosomes 1, 2, 3, 5, 6, 7, 8, 9, 10, 11, 14, 15, 18 and 20.

5. Pray that God would heal the regions of the chromosomes influencing diabetes. Pray for regions IDDM1 – IDDM18.

6. Pray that God would heal each gene involved in diabetes and restore it to the normal purpose God intended before the foundation of the earth.

7. Pray that God would heal the HLA genes that encode immune response proteins located on chromosome 6p21.3. Pray also that God would heal the genes DQB1 and DRB1 both located on chromosome 6p21.3

8. Pray that God would heal the non-HLA genes, specifically the insulin gene located on region IDDM2 located on chromosome 11p15.5

9. Pray that God would heal the genes on region IDDM4 on Chromosome 11q13.3-11q13.4 which include ZFM1, FADD and LRP5.

10. Pray that God would heal the genes on region IDDM5 on chromosome 6q25.2 – 6q25.3 which include SOD2.

11. Pray that God would heal the genes on region IDDM6 on chromosome 18q21 which include ZNF236.

12. Pray that God would heal the genes on region IDDM7 on chromosome 2q37 which include NEUROD1 and IGRP.

13. Pray the God would heal the genes on region IDDM10 on chromosome 10p11.23 which include GAD2 and GAD65.

14. Pray that God would heal the genes on region IDDM11 on chromosome 14q31 which include ENSA, KIR, ABCC8 and SEL1L.

15. Pray that God would heal the genes on region IDDM12 on chromosome 2q33 which include CTLA4, CD28 and ICOS.

16. Pray that God would heal the genes on region IDDM18 on chromosome 5q34 which include ILB12, IL-12 and IL-12p40.

17. Pray the God would heal the genes involved in type 2 diabetes which include CAPN10 located on chromosome 2q37.3, HNF4A located on Chromosome 20q12-20q13.1 , GCGR located on chromosome 17q25, GLUT2 located on chromosome 3, HNF4A located on chromosome 20q12 – 20q13.1, and ABCC8 located on chromosome 11p15.1.

18. Pray that God would heal and restore the cardiovascular system, the eyes, the kidneys, the nerves and other organ system or cells that have been damaged by diabetes.

19. Thank God for restoring function of the genes and chromosomes we have listed.

20. Thank God for healing and restoring the function of the genes and chromosomes involved in diabetes that we don't know about. We thank you God that You are our creator, know us intimately and You know each and every defect down to the base pair of our genome structure that needs restoration. AMEN

Prayer for Breast Cancer

1. Have the person repent because of the sins of her ancestors, especially the sins of conflict and bitterness between the other females in the family, mother, sister, or mother-in-law, that allowed an iniquitous pattern to be passed down through her generations. Have her forgive her ancestors for passing that iniquitous pattern down and for any damage it did to cause a genetic based disorder. Have her repent of her own sins as well.

2. Lord I pray for the healing of all breast tissue that has been damaged because of cancer.

3. Lord, I curse any rebellious cells and command them to dry up and die.

4. Lord I ask that you restore normal cellular function of the breasts and any structures where the cancer may have spread or there has been metastasis.

5. Lord I pray for healing and restoration of the following genes and chromosomes whether they were inherited in a mutated state or became mutated in this individual.

6. I pray for the healing of any mutations in the tumor suppressor genes BRCA1 on Chromosome17q21 and BRCA2 on Chromosome 13q12-13q13 as well as BRAC3 and BRAC4 on Chromosome 13q21 and BRCD1 on 13pter – 13qter and I ask that you repair and restore them to function the way You created them to perform from the foundation of the earth.

7. Lord, I ask that you heal and restore the following genes and chromosomes whether they were passed down in a mutated state or became mutated in this individual.

HSPCA

BCAR2

BCAR3 on Chromosome 1p22.1 - 1p21.3

BCAS2 on Chromosome 1p21-1p13.3

GSTM1 on Chromosome 1p13.3

MUC1 on Chromosome 1q21

S100A4 on Chromosome 1q21

KISS1 on Chromosome 1q32

CYP1B1 on Chromosome 2p22-p21

SRD5A2 on Chromosome 2p23

BIN1 on Chromosome 2q14

BARD1 on Chromosome 2q34-q35

TGFBR2 on Chromosome 3p22

RARB on Chromosome 3p24

EIF4E on Chromosome 4q21-q25

HSPCB on Chromosome 6p12

TFAP2A on Chromosome 6p12

NOTCH 4 on Chromosome 6p21.3

TFAP2A on Chromosome 6p24

LIBC on Chromosome 6q22

TPD52L1 on Chromosome 6q22-q23

ESR1 on Chromosome 6q25.1

AMPH on Chromosome 7p14-p13

IL6 on Chromosome 7p21

HSPB1 on Chromosome 7q

TPD52 on Chromosome 8q21

TPD52 on Chromosome 8q21

EIF3S6 on Chromosome 8q22-q23

MYC on Chromosome 8q24.12-q24.23

BAG1 on Chromosome 9p12

CDKN2A on Chromosome 9p21

SNCG on Chromosome 10q23.2 – q23.3

PLAU on Chromosome 10q24

CYP17 on Chromosome 10q24.3

MK167 on Chromosome 10q25-qter

STIP1 on Chromosome 11

TSG101 on Chromosome 11p15.2 – 15.1

HRAS on Chromosome 11p15.5

IGF2 on Chromosome 11p15.5

CTSD on Chromosome 11p15.5

SLC22A1L on Chromosome 11p15.5

CD44 on Chromosome 11pter-p13

EMS1 on Chromosome 11q13

CCND1 on Chromosome 11q13

GSTP1 on Chromosome 11q13

ATM on Chromosome 11q22.3

CDKN1B on Chromosome 12p13

CD9 on Chromosome 12p13

ERBB3 on Chromosome 12q13

IGF1 on Chromosome 12q22-q24.1

RB1 on Chromosome 13q14.2

EFNB2 on Chromosome 13q33

SR2 on Chromosome 14q

CYP19 on Chromosome 15q21.1

CYP1A1 on Chromosome 15q22-q24

CSK on Chromosome 15q23-q25

IGF1R on Chromosome 15q25-q26

MMP2 on Chromosome 16q13

BCAR1 on Chromosome 16q23.1

MAP2K4 on Chromosome 17p11.2

TP53 on Chromosome 17p13.1

LASP1 on Chromosome 17q11-q21.3

ERBB2 on Chromosome 17q11.2-q12

TIMP2 on Chromosome 17q25

BIRC5 on Chromosome 17q25

PI5 on Chromosome 18q21.3

STK11 on Chromosome 19p13.3

KLK3 on Chromosome 19q13

PCNA on Chromosome 20p12

TFAP2C on Chromosome 20q13.2

BCAS1 on Chromosome 20q13.2-q13.3

TFF1 on Chromosome 21q22.3

PSEN2 on Chromosome 21q22.3

COMT on Chromosome 22q11.2

MMP11 on Chromosome 22q11.2

GSTT1 on Chromosome 22q11.23

CHEK2 on Chromosome 22q12.1

8. Lord please regulate, repair and restore genes FCF8 on Chromosome 10q24, ARHC on Chromosome 1p21 – p13 and ARHA on Chromosome 3p21.3 that are over-expressed in breast cancer. Please reduce the function of these genes to the expression that lines up with the way You created them to function from before the foundation of the earth.

9. Lord please regulate, repair and restore the gene COT on Chromosome 10p11.2 that is over-expressed and amplified in breast cancer. Please reduce the function of this gene to the expression that lines up with the way You created it to function from before the foundation of the earth.

10. Lord please regulate, repair and restore the gene ING1 on Chromosome 13q34 that is suppressed in breast cancer. Please increase

the function of this gene to the expression that lines up with the way You created it to function from before the foundation of the earth.

11. Lord please repair and restore any deletion on the short arm Chromosome 1 and restore all genes deleted from that area.

12. Lord I pray for gene p53 on Chromosome 17 and the p53 protein. I ask that You heal this gene and cause the protein to be produced and function properly as You intended from the foundation of the earth.

AMEN

Prayer for Li-Fraumeni Syndrome

This syndrome occurs when a person inherits only one functional copy of the p53 gene from his parents, he is then predisposed to cancer and usually develops several independent tumors in a variety of tissues in early adulthood. This condition is rare.

1. Have the person repent because of the sins of his ancestors especially the sins of bitterness and slander with the tongue that allowed an iniquitous pattern to be passed down through his generations. Have him forgive his ancestors for passing that iniquitous pattern down and for any damage it did to cause a genetic based disorder. Have him repent for his own sins as well.

2. Lord I pray for a creative miracle in this individual. I pray that you would create another functional copy of the gene p53 and set it in place where it belongs on Chromosome 17.

3. I pray that any mutant p53 protein be destroyed and healthy p53 protein be produced.

4. Lord I pray that any over-expression of the p53 transcription factor that has caused a malfunction of repair gene GADD45 or apoptotic inducer Bax be corrected and the proper function of these genes be restored.

5. Lord I pray that any tumors caused by this syndrome be dissolved and healthy tissue be restored.

AMEN

Prayer for Adenocarcinoma of the Lung

1. Have the person repent because of the sins of his ancestors especially the sins of bitterness and resentment that allowed an iniquitous pattern to be passed down through his generations. Have him forgive his ancestors for passing that iniquitous pattern down and for any damage it did to cause a genetic based disorder. Have him repent for his own sins as well.

2. Lord I ask that you heal and restore all lung tissue, airways, pleura, and mucous membrane, respiratory muscles, blood vessels and any damage that has been done to the respiratory system by adenocarcinoma of the lung.

3. I curse any rebellious cells and command them to dry up and die.

4. Lord I ask that you restore normal cellular function of the lung tissue and components of the respiratory tract, and any structures where the cancer may have spread or there has been metastasis.

5. Lord I ask that you heal and restore the following genes and chromosomes whether they were inherited in a mutated state or became mutated in this individual.

GSTM1 on Chromosome 1p13.3

MYCL1 on Chromosome 1p34.3

SLC2A1 on Chromosome 1p35-p31.3

TP73 on Chromosome 1p36

MUC1 on Chromosome 1q21

FHIT on Chromosome 3p14.2

DLEC1 on Chromosome 3p22-p21.3

SClC1 on Chromosome 3p23-p21

RARB on Chromosome 3p24

TERC on Chromosome 3q21-q28

ABCC5 on Chromosome 3q27

MUC4 on Chromosome 3q29

THBS2 on Chromosome 6q27

TNFRSF10B on Chromosome 8p22-p21

PDGFRL on Chromosome 8p22-p21.3

NAT1 on Chromosome 8p23.1-p21.3

PTEN on Chromosome 10q23.3

CYP2E on Chromosome 10q24.3-qter

DMBT1 on Chromosome 10q25.3-q26.1

MCMT on Chromosome 10q26

HRAS on Chromosome 11p15.5

SLC22A1L on Chromosome 11p15.5

PPP2R1B on Chromosome 11q22-q24

KRAS2 on Chromosome 12p12.1

CD9 on Chromosome 12p13

IGF1 on Chromosome 12q22-q24.1

RB1 on Chromosome 13q14.2

CYP1A1 on Chromosome 15q22-q24

MRP on Chromosome 16p13.1

RBL2 on Chromosome 16q12.2

CDH13 on Chromosome 16q24.2-q24.3

TP53 on Chromosome 17p13.1

ERBB2 on Chromosome 17q11.2-q12

TOP2A on Chromosome 17q21-q22

TIMP2 on Chromosome 17q25

BIRC5 on Chromosome 17q25

MADH2 on Chromosome 18q21

MADH4 on Chromosome 18q21.1

BCL2 on Chromosome 18q21.3

CYP2A6 on Chromosome 19q13.2

MMP11 on Chromosome 22q11.2

MIF on Chromosome 22q11.2

6. Lord I pray for gene SLC2A3 on Chromosome 12p13.3 that is over-expressed in Lung Cancer. Lord please reduce the function of this gene to the expression that lines up with the way You created it to function from before the foundation of the earth.

7. Lord I pray for gene CDKN2A on Chromosome 9p21 which is inactivated in Lung Cancer, Lord please restore and activate this gene to function in the manner You created it to function before the foundation of the earth.

8. Lord I pray for gene MYCN on Chromosome 2p24.1 and gene TNFRSF6B on Chromosome 20q13.3 that are amplified in lung cancer. Lord please regulate and restore the function on these genes to perform the way You intended them to function before the foundation of the earth.

9. I pray that any deletions in the short arm of chromosome 3 especially at 3p14, 3p21.3 and 3p25-p26 and the short arm of Chromosome 9 be repaired and restored. I pray that all genes deleted from those areas especially all tumor suppressor genes be restored to perform the way God intended before the foundation of the earth.

10. I especially pray for the gene RASSF1A on Chromosome 3p21.3 be restored and activated as a protector gene against Adenocarcinoma of the Lung.

11. Lord I pray that any amplification of the genes in the long arm of Chromosome 20 be regulated and restored to the function You intended for them to perform from before the foundation of the earth.

12. Lord I pray that any mutations of gene LKB1/STK11 on Chromosome 19p13.3 be corrected and restored to function the way You created it to perform before the foundation of the earth.

13. Lord I pray for gene p53 on Chromosome 17 and the p53 protein. I ask that You heal this gene and cause the protein to be produced and function properly as You intended from the foundation of the earth.

AMEN

Prayer for Colon Cancer

1. Have the person repent because of the sins of his ancestors especially the sins of unresolved bitterness, unresolved antagonism, frustration, anger and slander with the tongue that allowed an iniquitous pattern to be passed down through his generations. Have him forgive his ancestors for passing that iniquitous pattern down and for any damage it did to cause a genetic based disorder. Have him repent for his own sins as well.

2. Lord I pray for healing and restoration of any damaged tissue in the colon, rectum, or anywhere in the digestive tract.

3. I pray for healing and restoration of any muscle tissue, organ or cell that has wasted because of malnutrition.

4. I curse any rebellious cells and command them to dry up and die.

5. Lord I ask that you restore normal cellular function of the intestinal tract and any structures where the cancer may have spread or there has been metastasis.

6. Lord I pray for the healing and restoration of the following genes and chromosomes whether they were passed down in a mutated state or became mutated in this individual:

SDCCAG43 on Chromosome 9

MTHFR on Chromosome 1p36.3

MUCI on Chromosome 1q21

S100A4 on Chromosome 1q21

CRP on Chromosome 1q21-q23

PTSG2 on Chromosome 1q25.2-q25.3

REG1A on Chromosome 2p12

PMS1 on Chromosome 2q31-q33

TGFBR2 on Chromosome 3p22

CTTNB1 on Chromosome 3p22-p21.3

MCC on Chromosome 5q21

APC on Chromosome 5q21-q22

VEGF on Chromosome 6p12

PPARD on Chromosome 6p21.1-p21.2

CDKNIA on Chromosome 6p21.2

THBS2 on Chromosome 6q27

PMS2 on Chromosome 7p22

ABCB4 on Chromosome 7q21.1

TNFRSF10B on Chromosome 8p22-p21

BAI1 on Chromosome 8q21

CDKN2A on Chromosome 9p21

HRAS on Chromosome 11p15.5

IGF2 on Chromosome 11p15.5

CD44 on Chromosome 11pter-p13

PPP2R1B on Chromosome 11q22-q24

KRAS 2 on Chromosome 12p12.1

CDKN1B on Chromosome 12p13

IGF1 on Chromosome 12q22-q24.1

ALDH2 on Chromosome 12q24.2

SDCCAG1 on Chromosome 14q22

THBS1 on Chromosome 15q15

CSK on Chromosome 15q23-q25

MMP2 on Chromosome 16q13

TP53 on Chromosome 17p13.1

TOP2A on Chromosome 17q21-q22

AXIN2 on Chromosome 17q23-q24

BIRC5 on Chromosome 17q25

MADH2 on Chromosome 18q21

MADH4 on Chromosome 18q21.1

BCL2 on Chromosome 18q21.3

DCC on Chromosome 18q21.3

STK11 on Chromosome 19p13.3

AXL on Chromosome 19q13.1

BGP1 on Chromosome 19q13.2

CEACAM7 on Chromosome 19q13.2

BAX on Chromosome 19q13.3-13.4

PYGB on Chromosome 20p11.2-p11.1

MMP9 on Chromosome 20q11.2-q13.1

SRC on Chromosome 20q12-q13

TNFRSF6B on Chromosome 20q13.3

7. I pray that any deletions in the short arm of Chromosome 1 especially in the areas of 1p36.3, 1p35.1-p36.3 and 1p34.2-p35 and the short arm of Chromosome 8 be repaired and restored. I pray for all genes deleted from those areas including all tumor suppressor genes especially the LPH gene on Chromosome 8p22 and NEFL gene on Chromosome 8p21 be restored to perform the way God intended before the foundation of the earth.

8. Lord I pray that any mutation to gene MSH6 on Chromosome 2p16, gene MSH2 on Chromosome 2p22-p21 and gene MLH1 on Chromosome 3p21.3 be corrected and their function as repair genes be restored to the purpose that You created for them to perform before the foundation of the earth.

9. Lord I pray that any allelic loss on the long arm of Chromosome 18 be restored and repaired.

10. Lord I pray for gene p53 on Chromosome 17 and the p53 protein. I ask that You heal this gene and cause the protein to be produced and function properly as You intended from the foundation of the earth.

AMEN

Prayer for Dysautonomia

Dysautonomia is a dysfunction of the autonomic nervous system. A number of neurological disorders may be caused by Dysautonomia including postural orthostatic tachycardia syndrome (POTS), neurocardiogenic syncope, mitral valve prolapse, pure autonomic failure, multiple system atrophy (Shy-Drager Syndrome) to name a few. The disorder disturbs cells in the autonomic nervous system, which controls involuntary actions such as digestion, breathing, production of tears, and the regulation of blood pressure and body temperature. It also affects the sensory nervous system, which controls activities related to the senses, such as taste and the perception of pain, heat and cold.

1. Have the person repent because of the sins of his ancestors, especially the sins of fear, anxiety, stress, tension, panic, panic attacks, phobias, rages, anger and aggression that allowed an iniquitous pattern to be passed down through his generations. Have him forgive his ancestors for passing that iniquitous pattern down and for any damage it did to cause a genetic based disorder. Have him repent of his own sins as well.

2. Lord I ask that you heal every symptom that has been caused by this disorder. I ask that you heal any damage done to any organ that has been affected and restore it to the function You created it to perform before the creation of the earth.

3. Lord I ask that you heal the hypothalamus and cause it to integrate the autonomic nervous system and the endocrine system properly.

4. Lord I ask that you heal and restore the cells in the nervous system that have been damaged and cause the body to produce healthy cells.

5. Lord I ask that you correct mutations in the IKBKAP gene located on Chromosome 9q31, remove the duplication of the mutated gene which causes part of it to be skipped when it is copied for production of the IKAP protein, and restore it to its normal function.

6. Lord I ask you to heal gene IKBKAP causing the proper

production and function of IKAP protein to allow muscle and nerve fibers and synapses to perform as You intended from the foundation of the earth.

7. Lord I ask that you correct all transmissions on Chromosome 9 so that this individuals nerves, muscle fibers and synapses perform in the way You intended from the foundation of the earth

AMEN

About Jubilee Resources International

God's commission for Jubilee Resources International is based on Ezekiel 33:1-9, and Luke 4:18-21. According to the Bible, Jubilee years were times of restitution. Debts were cancelled, slaves set free, families reunited and lost or forfeited inheritances restored. Every year was prophetic of the ministry of Jesus Christ. The Jubilee was proclaimed on the basis of the work of the High Priest on the Day of Atonement - so Jesus Christ's liberating ministry is founded on His atoning work. Jesus began His public ministry by reading the passage from the prophet Isaiah (Luke 4:18-21). All the liberties of the Jubilee year are now available to us through the redemptive work of Jesus Christ at Calvary, and we all have the responsibility to preach this Gospel of Redemption and Restoration to full Relationship with Yahweh/Father God. When Yeshua/Jesus Christ returns, God's people will be totally free from all sin, sickness and disease, death and curse. The Biblical Jubilee will then be fully realized.

Resources in print book, eBook, audio & video formats are available in English, with paper & eBooks in Spanish, German, French, Italian, Portuguese-Brazil, Polish, Ukrainian, Russian, Dutch, Swedish, Danish, Norwegian, Finnish, Hungarian, Romanian, Slovak, Czech, Greek, Bulgarian, Estonian, Latvian, Lithuanian, Afrikaans, Malaysian, Indonesian & Tagalog, with other languages pending.

Additional Resources Available from

Jubilee Resources International Inc.

www.jubileeresources.org

Plus comprehensive range of free tracts to download

Dealing with Curses & Generational Iniquities. This teaching offers hope for all Christians that they can be released into the blessings of God and forever leave behind iniquities and curses that have kept them captive, perhaps their whole families for generations. This explains the twelve major curses that people may have operating in their families, and what to do about them. It also includes new material on the curses over Scottish, English, Irish, Welsh and Scandinavian people, plus many other national and ethnic groups. This teaching has been taught in several nations with much fruit for personal, family and community liberty. Best Seller *Book, E-book, MP4*

Dealing with Demons: *Insights into evil spiritual influences.* This popular teaching provides outstanding insights regarding evil spiritual influences that exist in the world in which we live today, and then goes further to show us what to do about it. Best Seller *Book, E-book, MP4*

Insights into Martial Arts, Tai Ch'i TM & Yoga. Much of the western world has seen an explosion of these practices. For many, their involvement has became close to a religion, adopting belief systems, mind sets and practises inconsistent with the teachings of the Bible. Best Seller *Book, E-book, MP4*

Treated or Tricked - Alternative Health Therapies Diagnosed. Many people are now trying Alternative Health Therapies. This book explains the various medical & spiritual healing methods; investigates whether the "Energy/Life Force" is scientific or spiritual; and describes almost 80 different Alternative Therapies, from Aromatherapy to Zone therapies. Also examines reasons why some are not healed & how to overcome these failures Biblically. Co-authored with Dr. Badu Bediako, (former Assoc. Professor of BioChemistry.) Best Seller *Book, E-book, MP4*

Biblical Healing Training Manual. This thorough examination of Biblical physical healing is the result of many years of experience as well as training under some of the world's best Bible teachers. There are many "How To's", practical prayer and ministry guidelines, reasons why some aren't healed, and what we can do about them, etc. Hundreds have been healed, & many congregations have been empowered to commence regular Healing services with Christ-glorifying results. Best Seller *Book, E-book, MP4*

How to Minister to Change Lives and Communities. This comprehensive & practical training manual is for those who want to do effective ministry. This can include end-of-service and small-group ministry. Topics include Understanding the Spiritual Realm; Empowerment to Serve; Healing of the Body, & the Soul; Deeper Ministry by appointment & referral; & Biblical blessings to release identity and destiny. Best Seller, *Book, E-book, MP4*

Made in the USA
Monee, IL
04 November 2026

67375616R00036